EKG in a Heartbeat

A Pocket Guide for Busy Healthcare Professionals

Karen M. Ellis, RN, CCRN

Prentice Hall

Upper Saddle River, NJ 07458

Library of Congress Cataloging-in-Publication Data

Ellis, Karen.
    EKG in a heartbeat : a pocket guide for busy healthcare
professionals / by Karen Ellis.
        p. cm.
    ISBN 0-13-061440-8
    1. Electrocardiography–Handbooks, manuals, etc.   I. Title: EKG
in a heartbeat.   II. Title.
    [DNLM: 1. Electrocardiography–Handbooks. WG 39 E47e 2001]
RC683.5.E5 E44 2001
616.1'207547–dc21

                                                    2001034361

Pearson Education LTD.
Pearson Education Australia PTY, Limited
Pearson Education Singapore, Pte. Ltd
Pearson Education North Asia Ltd
Pearson Education Canada, Ltd.
Pearson Educación de Mexico, S.A. de C.V.
Pearson Education–Japan
Pearson Education Malaysia, Pte. Ltd

Publisher: Julie Alexander
Executive Assistant & Supervisor: Regina Bruno
Acquisitions Editor: Mark Cohen
Editorial Assistant: Melissa Kerian
Managing Editor: Patrick Walsh
Production Management/Composition Electronic Art Creation: North Market Street Graphics
Production Editor: North Market Street Graphics
Interior Design: North Market Street Graphics
Director of Manufacturing and Production: Bruce Johnson
Manufacturing Buyer: Ilene Sanford
Creative Director: Cheryl Asherman
Design Coordinator: Maria Guglielmo
Marketing Manager: David Hough
Printer/Binder: Banta Company, Harrisonburg, VA
Cover Design: Joseph DePinho

Contents

Acknowledgments

To my family—Lee, Jason, Mark, and Matthew—for their patience during the preparation of this project.

To my editor Mark Cohen and editorial assistant Melissa Kerian for guiding me through this process and being supportive of this effort.

To my EKG students at Delgado Community College and my coworkers at Touro Infirmary in New Orleans for their support of and enthusiasm for this effort.

Introduction

You're busy. And you've got a mountain of information to master as part of your position (or your desired position) in healthcare. So you could really use a quick reference on EKG interpretation. You need a pocket guide.

But which one? There are lots of them out there.

Unlike some pocket guides, which are essentially miniature versions of textbooks a few hundred pages long, this pocket guide has the pertinent facts you need to help you read rhythm strips and 12-lead EKGs, **but it doesn't take hundreds of pages to say it.** Fast, accurate, and to the point. With time at a premium, you can't afford to waste precious minutes wading through tons of information that you *don't* need in order to find the one piece of information you *do* need.

A word of caution, however. This book is not intended as an elementary text on electrocardiography. It is a "cut-to-the-chase-what-do-I-need-to-know-this-second" kind of book. It presumes at least a basic knowledge of EKG principles. If you want a comprehensive EKG textbook, consider my textbook *EKG Plain and Simple*.

Contained within this pocket guide are algorithms for rhythm interpretation, axis, hypertrophy, bundle branch blocks and hemiblocks, and myocardial infarct localization as well as examples of the various rhythms and types of MIs. There is also a 12-lead interpretation checklist so you know exactly what to look for when you examine EKGs.

And there's a lot more.

Written in plain English, this pocket guide is a very informal, friendly aid to EKG interpretation.

Hope you find it helpful.

Sincerely,

Karen Ellis, RN, CCRN

How to Analyze a Rhythm Strip

Rhythm Interpretation Words of Wisdom

- All matching upright P waves are sinus P waves until proven otherwise.

- Sinus rhythms must have an atrial rate less than or equal to 160 **in a resting adult.**

- On rhythms with two different-shaped P waves, one of those Ps is *probably* sinus. On rhythms with three or more different-shaped Ps, one cannot be sure if *any* are sinus Ps.

- All wide QRS beats without preceding P waves are ventricular until proven otherwise.

- All irregular rhythms are atrial fibrillation until proven otherwise.

- If the QRS complexes look alike, the T waves that follow them should also look alike. A T wave that suddenly changes shape when the QRS complexes don't is hiding a P wave inside it.

- The most common cause of an unexplained pause is a nonconducted PAC.

- Absence of conduction is not necessarily because of a block. Block implies a pathologic process. Absence of conduction may be simply due to refractoriness, a normal physiologic process.

Rhythm Interpretation Steps

1. Are there QRS complexes?
   - If there are no QRS complexes, the rhythm is either asystole, ventricular asystole, or ventricular fibrillation. All other rhythms have QRS complexes.

How to Analyze a Rhythm Strip (cont'd)

- If there are QRSs, are they the same shape, or does the shape vary?
- If there are no QRSs, skip to question 4.

2. Is the rhythm regular, regular but interrupted, or irregular?
   - Compare the R-R intervals (the distance between consecutive QRSs).

3. What is the heart rate?
   - If the heart rate is greater than 100, the patient is said to have a **tachycardia.**
   - If the heart rate is less than 60, the patient has a **bradycardia.**

4. Are there P waves?
   - If so, what is their relationship to the QRS? In other words, are the Ps always in the same place relative to the QRS, or are the Ps in different places with each beat?
   - Are any Ps not followed by a QRS?
   - Are the Ps all the same shape, or does the shape vary?
   - Is the P-P interval regular?

5. What are the PR, QRS, and QT intervals?
   - Are the intervals within normal limits, or are they too short or too long?
   - Are the intervals constant, or do they vary?

How to Determine the Regularity of a Rhythm

There are three basic types of regularity:

1. **Regular.** R-R intervals are constant and vary only by one or two little blocks. On the following strip, the R-R intervals are all about 20 little blocks apart. The rhythm is regular.

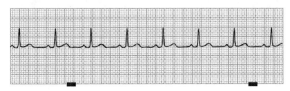

2. **Regular but interrupted.** This is a regular rhythm interrupted by premature beats or pauses. Strip A shows a regular rhythm interrupted by a premature beat (indicated by the dot) and the short pause that normally follows it. Strip B shows a regular rhythm interrupted by a pause.

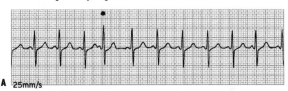

A 25mm/s

B

How to Determine the Regularity of a Rhythm (cont'd)

3. **Irregular.** R-R intervals vary throughout the strip.

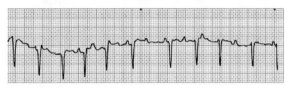

Rhythm Regularity Summary

The following table points out the type of regularity of each rhythm. *Only rhythms with QRS complexes are shown here.*

Origin of Rhythm	Regular	Regular but Interrupted	Irregular
Sinus	• Sinus rhythm • Sinus bradycardia • Sinus tachycardia	• Sinus arrest • Sinus pause • Sinus exit block	• Sinus arrhythmia
Atrial	• SVT • Atrial tachycardia (nonparoxysmal) • Atrial flutter (if the conduction ratio is constant) • 2:1 atrial tachycardia	• PACs • Paroxysmal atrial tachycardia	• Wandering atrial pacemaker • Multifocal atrial tachycardia • Atrial fibrillation • Atrial flutter (if the conduction ratio varies)
Junctional	• Junctional bradycardia • Junctional rhythm • Accelerated junctional rhythm • Junctional tachycardia	• PJCs	• None
Ventricular	• Idioventricular rhythm • Accelerated idioventricular rhythm • Ventricular tachycardia • Ventricular flutter • Paced rhythm	• PVCs • Paced beats	• Agonal rhythm • Torsades de pointes
AV blocks	• First-degree AV block (if the underlying rhythm is regular) • 2:1 AV block • Type II second-degree AV block (if the conduction ratio is constant and it does not interrupt another rhythm) • Third-degree AV block	• Type II second-degree AV block (if it interrupts another rhythm) • Type I second-degree AV block (is usually irregular but may look RBI at times)	• First-degree AV block (if the underlying rhythm is irregular) • Type I second-degree AV block • Type II second-degree AV block (if the conduction ratio varies)

How to Calculate Heart Rate

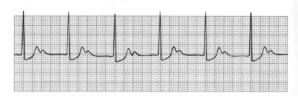

1. Count the number of big blocks between consecutive QRS complexes and divide into 300. On the sample strip, you'll note the QRSs are all five big blocks apart. $300 \div 5 = 60$.

or

2. Count the number of little blocks between consecutive QRS complexes and divide into 1,500. On the sample strip, the QRSs are all 25 little blocks apart. $1,500 \div 25 = 60$.

or

3. Count the number of QRS complexes on a 6-second strip and multiply by 10. On the sample, there are six QRS complexes on this 6-second strip, so the **mean (average) heart rate** is 60.

Regularity-Based Heart Rate Calculation	
Rhythm Regularity	**Kind of Heart Rate to Calculate**
Regular	One heart rate, using big or little block method
Regular but interrupted by premature beats	One heart rate (ignoring premature beats)
Regular but interrupted by pauses	Range slowest to fastest, plus mean rate
Irregular	Range slowest to fastest, plus mean rate

Heart Rate Chart

Count the number of little blocks between QRS complexes and follow the dots to the HR.

Blocks	HR	Blocks	HR	Blocks	HR
1	1,500	21	71	41	37
2	750	22	68	42	36
3	500	23	65	43	35
4	375	24	62	44	34
5	300	25	60	45	33
6	250	26	58	46	33
7	214	27	56	47	32
8	187	28	54	48	31
9	167	29	52	49	31
10	150	30	50	50	30
11	137	31	48	51	29
12	125	32	47	52	29
13	115	33	45	53	28
14	107	34	44	54	28
15	100	35	43	55	27
16	94	36	42	56	27
17	88	37	41	57	26
18	83	38	39	58	26
19	79	39	38	59	25
20	75	40	37	60	25

How to Determine Intervals

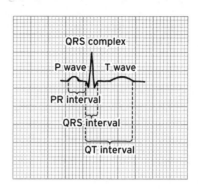

PR Interval

Count the number of little blocks between the beginning of the P wave and the beginning of the QRS complex. Multiply by 0.04 second. Normal PR interval is 0.12 to 0.20 second (between three and five little blocks).

QRS Interval

Count the number of little blocks between the beginning and end of the QRS complex. Multiply by 0.04 second. Normal QRS interval is <0.12 second (less than three little blocks wide).

QT Interval

Count the number of little blocks between the beginning of the QRS complex and the end of the T wave. Multiply by 0.04 second. Normal QT interval varies with the heart rate. At heart rates between 60 to 100, the QT interval should be less than half the R-R interval.

The Skinny on Sinus Rhythms

The sinus node is the acknowledged king of the conduction system's pacemaker cells. And there are only two ways for the sinus node king to relinquish its throne:

1. By illness or death, requiring someone to step in for it (escape)

2. By being overthrown by a subordinate (usurpation)

Though they can be irregular at times, sinus rhythms are, for the most part, notoriously regular. They're like the ticking of a clock–predictable and expected. The inherent rate of the sinus node is 60 to 100, but remember that this rate can go higher or lower if the sinus node is acted on by the sympathetic or parasympathetic nervous system. The individual's tolerance of these rhythms will depend in large part on the heart rate. Heart rates that are too fast or too slow can cause symptoms of decreased cardiac output.

Treatment is not needed unless symptoms develop. At that time, the goal is to return the heart rate to normal levels.

Sinus rhythms are the standard against which all other rhythms are compared. Since most of the rhythms you will see in real life will be sinus rhythms, you'll need a thorough understanding of them. Let's look at the criteria for sinus rhythms. *All these criteria must be met for the rhythm to be sinus in origin.*

The Skinny on Sinus Rhythms (cont'd)

- **Upright matching P waves followed by a QRS (P may be inverted in V₁)** *and*
- **PR intervals constant** *and*
- **Heart rate ≤ 160 at rest**

All matching upright P waves are considered sinus P waves until proven otherwise. The width and deflection of the QRS complex is irrelevant in determining whether a rhythm is sinus. The QRS may be narrow (<0.12 s) or wide (≥0.12 s), depending on the state of conduction through the bundle branches. The deflection of the QRS will depend on the lead in which the patient is being monitored.

Sinus Rhythms Pictorial

Sinus Rhythm

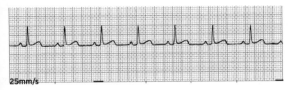

Criteria: Matching, usually upright P waves followed by a QRS, constant PR interval, HR 60 to 100

Sinus Bradycardia

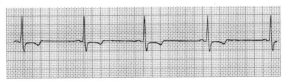

Criteria: Same as sinus rhythm, except HR < 60

Sinus Tachycardia

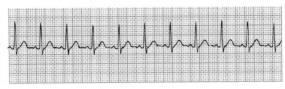

Criteria: Same as sinus rhythm, except HR > 100 (and ≤160 in a resting adult)

Sinus Rhythms Pictorial (cont'd)

Sinus Arrhythmia

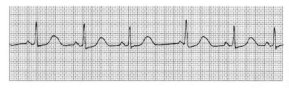

Criteria: Matching, usually upright Ps preceding QRSs, PR constant, HR irregular; the longest R-R interval exceeds the shortest by four little blocks or more.

Sinus Arrest

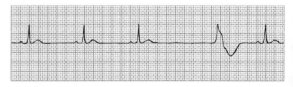

Criteria: The beat at the end of the pause is *not* a sinus beat. The pause interrupts a sinus rhythm of some sort.

Sinus Pause

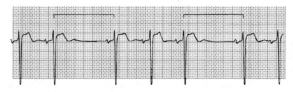

Criteria: The beat at the end of the pause is a sinus beat. The pause is not a multiple of the previous R-R intervals. The pause interrupts a sinus rhythm of some sort.

Sinus Rhythms Pictorial (cont'd)

Sinus Exit Block

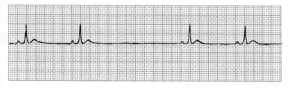

Criteria: The beat at the end of the pause is a sinus beat. The pause is a multiple of the previous R-R intervals. The pause interrupts a sinus rhythm of some sort.

Sick Sinus Syndrome

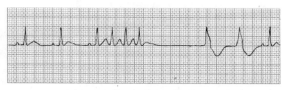

Criteria: Alternating tachyarrhythmias and bradyarrhythmias with pauses and escape beats, very irregular

The Skinny on Atrial Rhythms

The atrium is the pacemaker next in line below the sinus node. Though theoretically this positions it to escape if the sinus node fails (the inherent rate of the atrium is 60 to 80), the atrium does not often function in an escape role. In fact, atrial escape beats are very uncommon. The atria like to fire rapidly and are much more likely to become hyper and usurp control from the sinus node than to escape and fire slowly when the sinus node fails. Since atrial rhythms often result in very rapid heart rates, patients are often symptomatic.

Treatment is aimed at converting the rhythm back to sinus rhythm, or, if that is not possible, returning the heart rate to more normal levels.

Atrial rhythms are extremely variable in their presentation. Some rhythms have obvious P waves. Others have no Ps at all–instead, they have fibrillatory or flutter waves between the QRS complexes. Some atrial rhythms are regular and others are completely irregular, even chaotic. Though most atrial rhythms are rapid, a few are slower.

Unlike sinus rhythms, which have a common set of criteria, atrial rhythms have multiple and variable possible criteria. If the rhythm or beat in question meets *any* of these criteria, it is atrial in origin. Let's look at these criteria now:

The Skinny on Atrial Rhythms
(cont'd)

- Matching upright Ps, atrial rate > 160 at rest *or*
- No Ps at all; wavy or sawtooth baseline between QRSs present instead *or*
- P waves of ≥ three different shapes *or*
- Premature abnormal P wave (with or without QRS) interrupting another rhythm, *or*
- Heart rate ≥ 130, rhythm regular, P waves not discernible (may be present, but can't be sure)

Atrial Rhythms Pictorial

Wandering Atrial Pacemaker

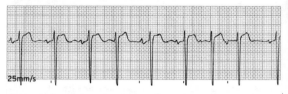

Criteria: Irregular rhythm with at least three different shapes of P waves, HR < 100

PACs

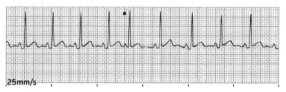

Criteria: Premature, abnormally shaped P wave followed by a QRS. PACs usually interrupt some sort of sinus rhythm.

Atrial Rhythms Pictorial (cont'd)

Nonconducted PAC

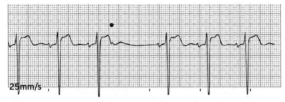

Criteria: Premature, abnormally shaped P wave *not* followed by a QRS. Nonconducted PACs usually interrupt a sinus rhythm of some sort.

Paroxysmal Atrial Tachycardia

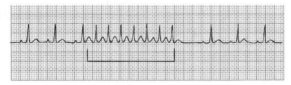

Criteria: This is a burst of atrial tachycardia that interrupts another rhythm (usually sinus). Atrial tachycardia's HR is 160 to 250, regular, with a narrow QRS.

Atrial Tachycardia with 2:1 Block

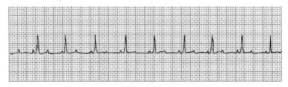

Criteria: Atrial rate 160 to 250 and regular, ventricular rate half the atrial rate

Atrial Rhythms Pictorial (cont'd)

Multifocal Atrial Tachycardia

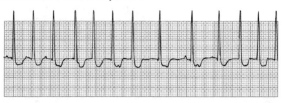

Criteria: Irregular rhythm with three or more different shapes of Ps, HR > 100. This is the same rhythm as wandering atrial pacemaker, but with a faster HR.

Atrial Flutter

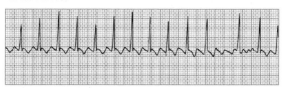

Criteria: Zigzag or sawtooth-shaped waves between the QRS complexes. There are no P waves. Flutter waves are all the same distance from each other.

Atrial Fibrillation

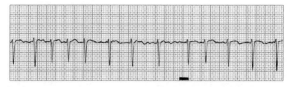

Criteria: Wavy or undulating baseline between QRS complexes. There are no P waves. Regularity is irregular.

Atrial Rhythms Pictorial (cont'd)

Supraventricular Tachycardia

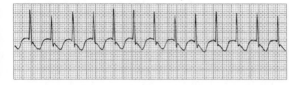

Criteria: Regular rhythm with narrow QRS complex and indistinguishable P waves, HR ≥ 130. The origin of the rhythm is unclear but is above the ventricle, as evidenced by the narrow QRS.

The Skinny on Junctional Rhythms

Junctional rhythms are seen less often than sinus or atrial rhythms. Though the inherent rate of the AV node is 40 to 60, the heart rate may actually go much faster or slower, and can result in symptoms. More normal heart rates are less likely to cause symptoms.

Treatment is aimed at alleviating the cause of the junctional rhythm. More active treatment is not usually necessary unless symptoms develop, at which time the goal is to return the sinus node to control or to return the heart rate to more normal levels.

Junctional rhythms are very easy to identify. Let's look at the criteria:

- **Regular rhythm or premature beat with narrow QRS and one of the following:**

  Absent P waves

  Inverted P waves following the QRS

  Inverted P waves with short PR interval preceding the QRS

Junctional Rhythms Pictorial

PJCs

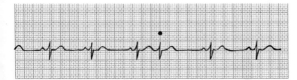

Criteria: Premature beat with inverted or absent P wave and a narrow QRS complex, interrupting a sinus rhythm of some sort. PR will be <0.12 second if inverted P precedes the QRS.

Junctional Bradycardia

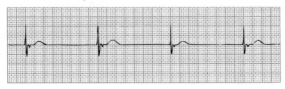

Criteria: Regular rhythm with a narrow QRS and inverted or absent P waves, HR < 40. PR will be <0.12 second if inverted P precedes the QRS.

Junctional Rhythm

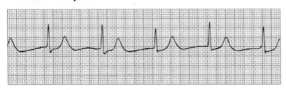

Criteria: Same as junctional bradycardia, except HR 40 to 60

Junctional Rhythms Pictorial (con't)

Accelerated Junctional Rhythm

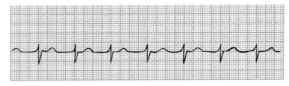

Criteria: Regular rhythm with narrow QRS and inverted or absent P waves, HR 60 to 100. PR will be <0.12 second if inverted P precedes the QRS.

Junctional Tachycardia

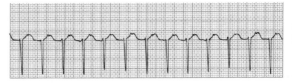

Criteria: Same as accelerated junctional rhythm, except HR > 100. PR will be <0.12 second if inverted P precedes the QRS.

The Skinny on Ventricular Rhythms

Ventricular rhythms are by far the most potentially lethal of all the rhythms. They therefore command great respect from healthcare personnel. Ventricular rhythms can result from escape (the inherent rate of the ventricle is 20 to 40) or usurpation, and can have a heart rate varying from 0 to over 250 beats per minute. Though some ventricular rhythms can be well tolerated, most will cause symptoms of decreased cardiac output, if not frank cardiac standstill.

Most ventricular rhythms respond well to medications. Oddly enough, however, some of the very medications used to treat ventricular rhythms can *cause* them in some circumstances. Some ventricular rhythms can only be treated by electric shock to the heart. And others, despite aggressive treatment, are usually lethal.

Ventricular beats have wide, bizarre QRS complexes. Some ventricular rhythms, however, have no QRS complexes at all. If the rhythm or beat in question meets *any* of the following criteria, it is ventricular in origin. Let's look at the criteria:

- **Wide QRS (>0.12 s) without preceding P wave** *or*
- **No QRS at all,** *or*
- **Premature, wide QRS beat without preceding P wave, interrupting another rhythm**

Ventricular Rhythms Pictorial

PVCs

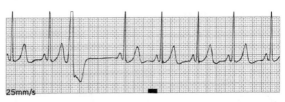

Criteria: Premature, wide QRS beat without preceding P wave, interrupting another rhythm (usually sinus)

Agonal Rhythm (Dying Heart)

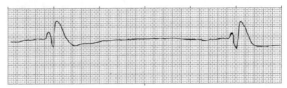

Criteria: Irregular rhythm with wide QRS and no preceding P wave, HR < 20

Idioventricular Rhythm

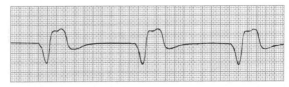

Criteria: Regular rhythm with wide QRS and no preceding P wave, HR 20 to 40

Ventricular Rhythms Pictorial
(cont'd)

Accelerated Idioventricular Rhythm

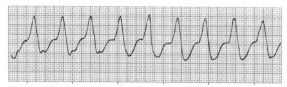

Criteria: Regular rhythm with wide QRS and no preceding P wave, HR 40 to 100

Ventricular Tachycardia

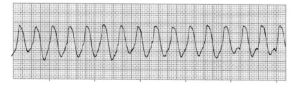

Criteria: Same as accelerated idioventricular rhythm, HR > 100

Torsades de Pointes

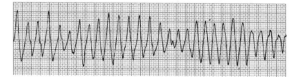

Criteria: Wide QRS without preceding P wave. QRS complexes rotate around an axis, pointing up and down, HR > 200. Torsades is recognized more by its characteristic oscillating pattern than by other criteria.

Ventricular Rhythms Pictorial
(cont'd)

Ventricular Flutter

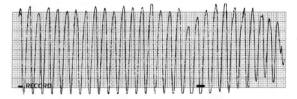

Criteria: Zigzag pattern of QRS complexes with HR 250 to 350

Ventricular Fibrillation

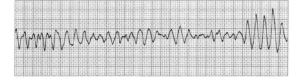

Criteria: No QRS complexes at all, just a wavy baseline looking like static

Asystole

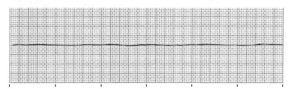

Criteria: No Ps or QRS complexes, flat line

Ventricular Rhythms Pictorial
(cont'd)

Ventricular Asystole

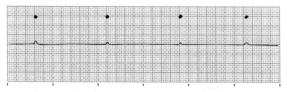

Criteria: No QRS complexes, P waves only

Ventricular Pacing

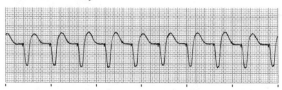

Criteria: Spike before each wide QRS complex

AV Sequential Pacing (Dual Chamber Pacing)

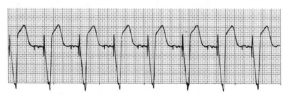

Criteria: Spike before the P wave and before the wide QRS

The Skinny on AV Blocks

In AV blocks, the underlying rhythm is sinus. The impulse is born in the sinus node and heads down the conduction pathway as usual. Thus the P waves are normal sinus P waves. Further down the conduction pathway, however, there is a roadblock. This can result in either a simple delay in impulse transmission or a complete or partial interruption in the conduction of sinus impulses to the ventricle. Heart rates can be normal or very slow, and symptoms may be present or absent. Treatment is aimed at increasing the heart rate and improving AV conduction.

There are two possible criteria for AV blocks. *If either of these criteria is met, there is an AV block.* Let's look at the criteria:

- **PR interval prolonged (>0.20 s) in some kind of sinus rhythm, *or***

- **Some Ps not followed by a QRS; P-P interval regular**

AV Blocks Pictorial

First-Degree AV Block

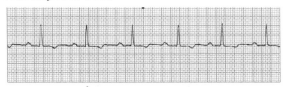

Criteria: Prolonged PR interval (>0.20 s) in a sinus rhythm of some sort

Type I Second-Degree AV Block (Wenckebach)

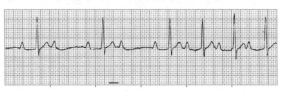

Criteria: P-P regular, PR interval varies, R-R interval varies. PR intervals gradually prolong until one P is not followed by a QRS.

Type II Second-Degree AV Block

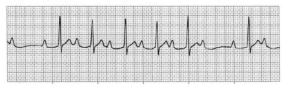

Criteria: P-P regular, PR interval constant on the conducted beats, some Ps not followed by a QRS

AV Blocks Pictorial (con't)

2:1 AV Block

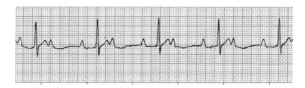

Criteria: P-P regular, R-R regular, PR interval regular. Only every other P wave is followed by a QRS.

Third-Degree AV Block (Complete Heart Block)

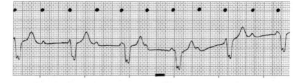

Criteria: P-P regular, R-R regular, PR intervals vary. Atrial rate is faster than ventricular rate. Some Ps are not followed by a QRS. There is complete AV dissociation. None of the P waves is associated with the QRS complexes, even though at times there may appear to be a relationship.

Main Algorithm for EKG Rhythm Interpretation

This algorithm is designed to point you to the secondary algorithms that will then pinpoint the rhythm. Here are some rules to get you started:

1. All matching upright P waves are sinus Ps until proven otherwise. Sinus rhythms have an atrial rate ≤160 at rest.
2. On rhythms with two different-shaped P waves, one of those Ps is *probably* sinus; on rhythms with three or more different-shaped Ps, one cannot be sure if *any* are sinus Ps.

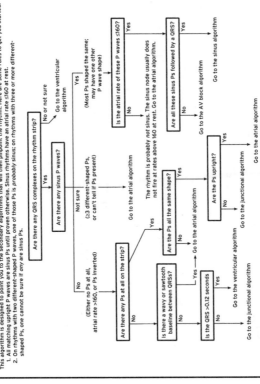

Sinus Algorithm

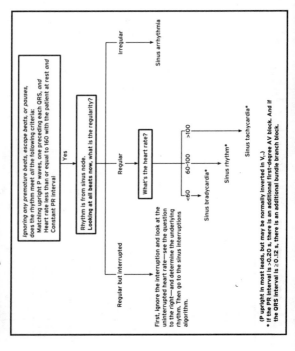

Ignoring any premature beats, escape beats, or pauses, does the rhythm meet *all* the following criteria:
- Matching upright P waves, one preceding each QRS, *and*
- Heart rate less than or equal to 160 with the patient at rest *and*
- Constant PR interval

Yes

Rhythm is from sinus node.
Looking at all beats now, what is the regularity?

Regular but interrupted

First, ignore the interruption and look at the uninterrupted heart rate—see the question to the right—and determine the underlying rhythm. Then go to the sinus interruptions algorithm.

Regular

What's the heart rate?

<60	60-100	>100
Sinus bradycardia*	Sinus rhythm*	Sinus tachycardia*

Irregular

Sinus arrhythmia

(P upright in most leads, but may be normally inverted in V₁.)

* If the PR interval is >0.20 s, there is an additional first-degree AV block. And if the QRS interval is ≥0.12 s, there is an additional bundle branch block.

Sinus Interruptions Algorithm

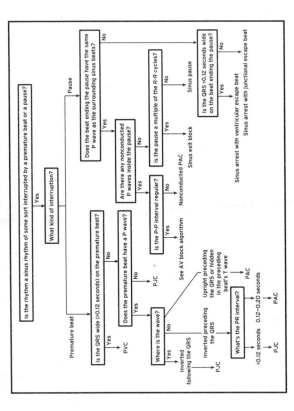

Is the rhythm a sinus rhythm of some sort interrupted by a premature beat or a pause?

Yes

What kind of interruption?

Premature beat

Is the QRS wide (>0.12 seconds) on the premature beat?

Yes → **PVC**

No → Does the premature beat have a P wave?

No → **PJC**

Yes → See AV block algorithm

Where is the wave?

Inverted following the QRS → **PJC**

Inverted preceding the QRS → **PJC**

Upright preceding the QRS or hidden in the preceding beat's T wave → **PAC**

What's the PR interval?

<0.12 seconds → **PJC**

0.12–0.20 seconds → **PAC**

Pause

Does the beat ending the pause have the same P wave as the surrounding sinus beats?

Yes → Are there any nonconducted P waves inside the pause?

Yes → Is the P-P interval regular?

Yes → **Sinus exit block**

No → **Nonconducted PAC**

No → Is the pause a multiple of the R-R cycles?

Yes → **Sinus block**

No → **Sinus pause**

No → Is the QRS >0.12 seconds wide on the beat ending the pause?

Yes → **Sinus arrest with ventricular escape beat**

No → **Sinus arrest with junctional escape beat**

33

Atrial Algorithm

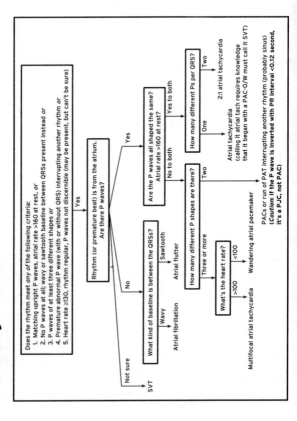

Does the rhythm meet *any* of the following criteria:
1. Matching upright P waves, atrial rate >160 at rest, or
2. No P waves at all; wavy or sawtooth baseline between QRSs present instead or
3. P waves of at least three different shapes or
4. Premature abnormal P wave (with or without QRS) interrupting another rhythm or
5. Heart rate ≥130, rhythm regular, P waves not discernible (may be present, but can't be sure)

Yes

Rhythm (or premature beat) is from the atrium.
Are there P waves?

Yes

Are the P waves all shaped the same?
Atrial rate >160 at rest?

Yes to both

How many different Ps per QRS?

One → Atrial tachycardia
(calling it atrial tach requires knowledge that it began with a PAC-O/W must call it SVT)

Two → 2:1 atrial tachycardia

No to both

How many different P shapes are there?

Two → PACs or run of PAT interrupting another rhythm (probably sinus)
(*Caution:* if the P wave is inverted with PR interval <0.12 second, it's a PJC, not PAC)

No

What kind of baseline is between the QRSs?

Wavy → Atrial fibrillation

Sawtooth → Atrial flutter

How many different P shapes are there?

Three or more → What's the heart rate?

<100 → Wandering atrial pacemaker

>100 → Multifocal atrial tachycardia

Not sure

SVT

34

Junctional Algorithm

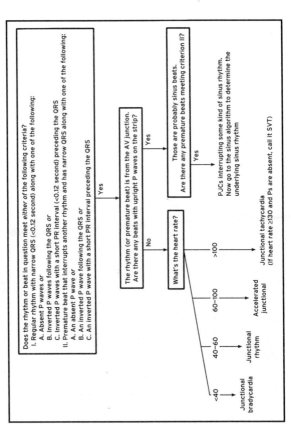

Does the rhythm or beat in question meet *either* of the following criteria?

I. Regular rhythm with narrow QRS (<0.12 second) along with one of the following:
    A. Absent P waves *or*
    B. Inverted P waves following the QRS *or*
    C. Inverted P waves with a short PR interval (<0.12 second) preceding the QRS

II. Premature beat that interrupts another rhythm and has narrow QRS along with one of the following:
    A. An absent P wave *or*
    B. An inverted P wave following the QRS *or*
    C. An inverted P wave with a short PR interval preceding the QRS

Yes

The rhythm (or premature beat) is from the AV junction.
Are there any beats with upright P waves on the strip?

No → What's the heart rate?

Yes → Those are probably sinus beats.
Are there any premature beats meeting criterion II?

Yes → PJCs interrupting some kind of sinus rhythm.
Now go to the sinus algorithm to determine the underlying sinus rhythm

What's the heart rate?

<40	40–60	60–100	>100
Junctional bradycardia	Junctional rhythm	Accelerated junctional	Junctional tachycardia (If heart rate ≥130 and Ps are absent, call it SVT)

Ventricular Algorithm

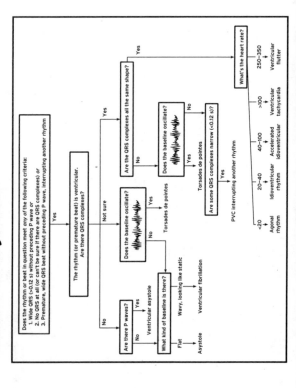

Does the rhythm or beat in question meet any of the following criteria:
1. Wide QRS (>0.12 s) without preceding P wave or
2. No QRS at all (or can't be sure if there are QRS complexes) or
3. Premature, wide QRS beat without preceding P wave, interrupting another rhythm

The rhythm (or premature beat) is ventricular.
Are there QRS complexes?

Yes → Are the QRS complexes all the same shape?

Yes → What's the heart rate?

<20	20–40	40–100	>100	250–350
Agonal rhythm	Idioventricular rhythm	Accelerated idioventricular rhythm	Ventricular tachycardia	Ventricular flutter

No → Does the baseline oscillate?

Yes → Torsades de pointes

No → Are some QRS complexes narrow (<0.12 s)?

Yes → PVC interrupting another rhythm

Not sure → Does the baseline oscillate?

No → Are there P waves?

Yes → Ventricular asystole

No → What kind of baseline is there?

Flat → Asystole

Wavy, looking like static → Ventricular fibrillation

Yes → Torsades de pointes

AV Block Algorithm

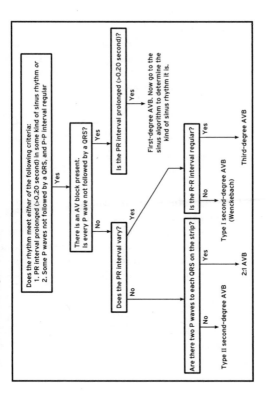

Does the rhythm meet *either of* the following criteria:
1. PR interval prolonged (>0.20 second) in some kind of sinus rhythm *or*
2. Some P waves not followed by a QRS, and P-P interval regular

Yes

There is an AV block present.
Is every P wave not followed by a QRS?

Yes

Is the PR interval prolonged (>0.20 second)?

Yes

First-degree AVB. Now go to the sinus algorithm to determine the kind of sinus rhythm it is.

No

Does the PR interval vary?

Yes

Is the R-R interval regular?

Yes

Third-degree AVB

No

Type I second-degree AVB (Wenckebach)

No

Are there two P waves to each QRS on the strip?

Yes

2:1 AVB

No

Type II second-degree AVB

Pacemaker Malfunctions

There are three basic types of pacemaker malfunctions:

1. **Failure to fire.** The pacemaker has failed to generate an impulse, perhaps because its battery is dead or the connecting wires are disrupted. Failure to fire is recognized by the absence of pacemaker spikes where there should have been.

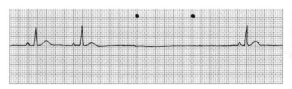

2. **Loss of capture.** The pacemaker has fired–there are pacemaker spikes–but there is no P wave or QRS following that spike. The pacemaker is not generating enough juice to cause the chamber to respond to the pacemaker's signal. Turning up the pacemaker's voltage often corrects this problem.

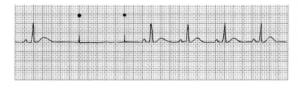

Pacemaker Malfunctions (con't)

3. **Undersensing.** The pacemaker does not sense ("see") the patient's own intrinsic beats, so it fires as if those beats weren't there. This results in paced beats or pacemaker spikes inside QRS complexes, in ST segments, or in other places too close to the intrinsic beats.

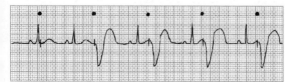

Lead Placement for a Standard 12-Lead EKG

Limb leads are on each arm and leg. Limb leads are leads I, II, III, aVR, aVL, and aVF. **Precordial (chest) leads** are located on the left chest. They are named V_1, V_2, V_3, V_4, V_5, and V_6.

Location of the Precordial Leads

V_1 Fourth intercostal space, right sternal border (abbreviated 4th ICS, RSB)

V_2 Fourth intercostal space, left sternal border (4th ICS, LSB)

V_3 Between V_2 and V_4

V_4 Fifth intercostal space, midclavicular line (5th ICS, MCL)

V_5 Fifth intercostal space, anterior axillary line (5th ICS, AAL)

V_6 Fifth intercostal space, midaxillary line (5th ICS, MAL)

Intercostal spaces are the spaces between the ribs. The fourth intercostal space is the space *below* the fourth rib; the fifth intercostal space is below the fifth rib, and so on. The **midclavicular line** is a line down from the middle of the clavicle (collarbone). The **anterior axillary line** is a line down from the front of the axilla (armpit). The **midaxillary line** is down from the middle of the axilla.

Lead Placement for a Standard 12-Lead EKG (con't)

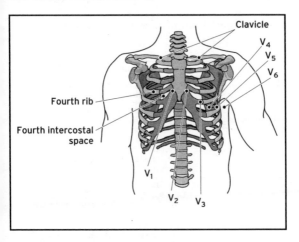

12-Lead EKG Interpretation in a Nutshell

Here's a breakdown of what you need to look for on every 12-lead EKG:

The Basics	Rhythm, rate, intervals (PR, QRS, QT)
Axis	Don't forget to put the + or − signs on the degree marking.
IVCDs (Intraventricular Conduction Defects)	RBBB = RSR' in V_1, QRS $\geq$ 0.12 s LBBB = QS or RS in V_1, monophasic R in V_6, QRS $\geq$ 0.12 s LAHB = Small Q in I, small R in III, left axis deviation LPHB = Small R in I, small Q in III, right axis deviation
Hypertrophy	RAE = Tall peaked P $\geq$ 2.5 mm in II or V_1 LAE = Notched P in II with 0.04 s between notches or P in any lead $\geq$ 0.11 s wide or biphasic P with terminal negative portion 1 mm wide and/or 1 mm deep RVH = R $\geq$ S in V_1, inverted T, right axis deviation LVH = S in V_1 + R in V_5 or $V_6 \geq$ 35 or R in aVL $\geq$ 11 mm or S in V_5 or $V_6 >$ 27 mm
Infarction/ Ischemia	Anterior MI = ST elevation and/or significant Q in V_1 to V_4 Inferior MI = ST elevation and/or significant Q in II, III, aVF Lateral MI = ST elevation and/or significant Q in I, aVL, V_5 to V_6 Anteroseptal MI = ST elevation and/or significant Q in V_1 to V_2 Extensive anterior (extensive anterior-lateral) = ST elevation and/or significant Q in I, aVL, V_1 to V_6 Posterior MI = Large R + upright T in V_1 to V_2; may also have ST depression Subendocardial = Widespread ST depression and T wave inversion in many leads Ischemia = Inverted T waves in any lead, as long as not BBB-related

12-Lead EKG Interpretation in a Nutshell (con't)

The Basics	Rhythm, rate, intervals (PR, QRS, QT)
Miscellaneous Effects	Digitalis effect = Sagging ST segments, prolonged PR interval
	Quinidine effect = Wide T waves causing prolonged QT interval
	Hyperkalemia = Tall, pointy, narrow T waves
	Severe hyperkalemia = Wide QRS complex
	Hypokalemia = Prominent U waves, flattened T waves
	Hypercalcemia = Shortened ST segment causing short QT interval
	Hypocalcemia = Prolonged ST segment causing prolonged QT interval

12-Lead EKG Interpretation Checklist

Use this checklist to document your findings on 12-lead EKGs.

The Basics

- Rhythm _____
- Rate _____
- Intervals   PR _____ QRS _____ QT _____

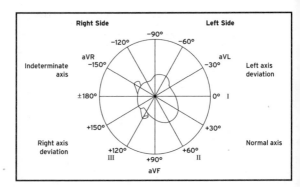

Axis

- Degree marking _____

Intraventricular Conduction Defects (IVCDs)

Check if present:

❏ RBBB   ❏ LBBB   ❏ LAHB   ❏ LPHB

12-Lead EKG Interpretation Checklist (con't)

Hypertrophy

Check if present:

❑ RAE ❑ LAE ❑ RVH ❑ LVH

Infarction

Check if present:

❑ Anterior MI

❑ Inferior MI

❑ Lateral MI

❑ Posterior MI

❑ Anteroseptal MI

❑ Extensive anterior (anterior-lateral) MI

❑ Subendocardial MI

❑ Ischemia

Miscellaneous Effects

Check if present:

❑ Hyperkalemia

❑ Severe hyperkalemia

❑ Hypokalemia

❑ Hypercalcemia

❑ Hypocalcemia

❑ Digitalis effect

❑ Quinidine effect

How to Calculate the Electrical Axis

There are four steps in calculating axis:

1. Determine the axis quadrant. Shade it in on the axis circle.
2. Find the lead with the most isoelectric QRS complexes.
3. Go to the perpendicular lead in the shaded quadrant.
4. Write down the degree marking at that lead. That's the axis.

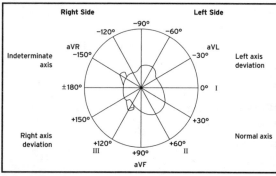

Axis circle

How to Determine the Axis Quadrant

Look at the QRS in leads I and aVF to determine the axis quadrant. Since lead I joins right arm and left arm, it tells us whether the axis is on the right or left side of the body. If lead I's QRS is positive, the axis will be on the positive side of the lead I line. That'll be on the left half of the circle (**the patient's left, not yours–imagine the axis circle on the patient's chest**). If lead I's QRS is negative, the axis will be on the negative side of lead I, which is on the right side of the circle. Shade in the right or left half of the circle.

aVF's positive pole is on the foot, so if aVF's QRS is positive, the axis will be on the lower half of the axis circle. A negative QRS in aVF will yield an axis on the top half of the circle. Shade in the top or bottom half of the circle.

By combining leads I and aVF, we find the axis quadrant. Following is a quick-and-dirty way of determining the axis quadrant, and therefore, axis deviation.

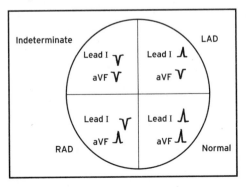

How to Determine the Axis Quadrant (con't)

If leads I and aVF are both positive, the axis is in the normal quadrant. If leads I and aVF are both negative, it's an indeterminate axis. If lead I is positive and aVF is negative, it's left axis deviation (LAD). If lead I is negative and aVF is positive, it's right axis deviation (RAD).

How to Determine the Most Isoelectric QRS Complex

The most isoelectric QRS complex is the one with the most equal positive and negative deflections. The axis will be on the lead perpendicular to this isoelectric lead. Examine leads I, II, III, aVR, aVL, and aVF to determine which is the most isoelectric.

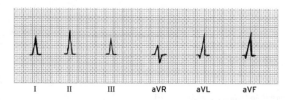

Which of these QRS complexes has the most dead-even positive and negative deflections? Usually, as on this example, it is easy to eyeball the most isoelectric. (It's aVR.)

Sometimes it's harder to tell which lead is the most isoelectric. In that case, for each lead, count the positive deflection in millimeters. Then count the negative deflection. Subtract the smaller number from the larger. This will tell how far off each lead is from being dead-even. The one that's the closest (with the smallest difference between positive and negative deflections) is the most isoelectric. See the following.

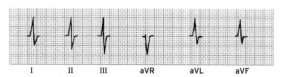

How to Determine the Most Isoelectric QRS Complex (con't)

Lead I is 10 mm positive and 5 mm negative, giving a difference of 5 mm.

Lead II is 10 mm positive and 7 mm negative, with a difference of 3 mm.

Lead III is 10 mm positive and 10 mm negative, with a difference of 0 mm.

aVR is 1 mm positive and 10 mm negative, with a difference of 9 mm.

aVL is 10 mm positive and 4 mm negative, with a difference of 6 mm.

aVF is 9 mm positive and 4 mm negative, with a difference of 5 mm.

Lead III has the smallest difference between positive and negative; therefore it is the most isoelectric.

The Perpendicular Rainbow

These connected leads are perpendicular to each other
(I and aVF, II and aVL, and III and aVR).

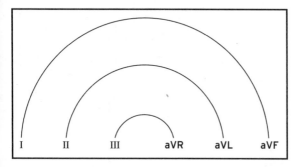

Axis Determination Algorithm

Here is a quick-and-dirty way to determine the axis when you're in a hurry. Just answer the questions and follow the arrows to the axis.

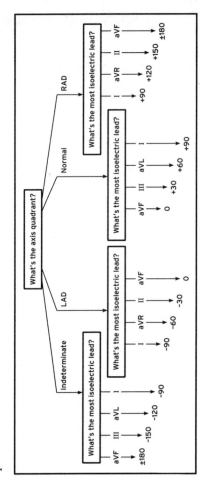

Bundle Branch Block/ Hemiblock Algorithm

Use this algorithm to determine if there is a BBB or hemiblock, or both, on the EKG. Just answer the questions and follow the arrows to the answer.

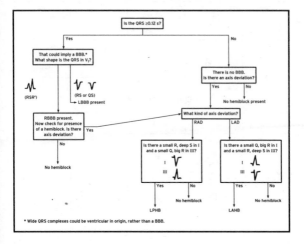

Criteria for Bundle Branch Blocks and Hemiblocks

Criteria for Bundle Branch Blocks

	QRS configuration in V_1	QRS configuration in V_6	QRS interval	T wave
RBBB	RSR′	QRS (wide terminal S)	≥0.12 s	Opposite the terminal QRS
LBBB	QS or RS	Monophasic R	≥0.12 s	Opposite the terminal QRS

Criteria for Hemiblocks

	Lead I	Lead III	QRS interval	Axis
LAHB	Small Q, taller R	Sm R, deeper S	<0.12 s	Left axis deviation
LPHB	Small R, deeper S	Sm Q, taller R	<0.12 s	Right axis deviation

Hypertrophy Algorithm

Hypertrophy can occur in the atria (more often referred to as atrial enlargement) or the ventricles. To assess for hypertrophy, we look at the size and shape of the P waves and the QRS complexes. This algorithm will point out atrial and ventricular hypertrophy. Just answer the questions and follow the arrows. *If none of the criteria are met, there is no hypertrophy.*

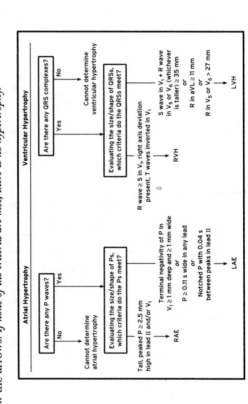

Evolution of an MI

Timeline	Age of MI	EKG Change	Implication
Immediately before the actual MI starts		T wave inversion	Cardiac tissue is ischemic, as evidenced by the newly inverted T waves.
Within hours after the MI's start	Acute	Marked ST elevation + upright T wave	Acute MI has begun, starting with myocardial injury.
Hours later	Acute	Significant Q + ST elevation + upright T	Some of the injured myocardial tissue has died, while other tissue remains injured.
Hours to a day or two later	Acute	Significant Q + less ST elevation + marked T inversion	Infarction is almost complete. Some injury and ischemia persist at the infarct edges.
Days to weeks later (in some cases this stage may last up to a year)	Age indeterminate	Significant Q + T wave inversion	Infarction is complete. Though there is no more ischemic tissue (it has either recovered or died), the T wave inversion persists.
Weeks, months, years later	Old	Significant Q only	The significant Q wave persists, signifying permanent tissue death.

How to Determine the Age of an MI

When an EKG is interpreted, the interpreter does not necessarily know the patient's clinical status and therefore must base determination of the MI's age on the indicative changes that are present on the EKG.

The age of an MI is determined as follows:

- An MI that has ST segment elevation is **acute** (one to two days old or less).

- An MI with significant Q waves, baseline (or almost back to baseline) ST segments, and inverted T waves is of **age indeterminate** (several days old, up to a year in some cases). Some authorities call this a **recent MI.**

- The MI with significant Q waves, baseline ST segments, and upright T waves is **old** (weeks to years old).

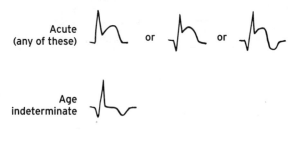

Acute (any of these)   or   or

Age indeterminate

Old

Infarction Squares

Each lead square is labeled with the wall of the heart at which it looks. When you analyze an EKG, note which leads have ST elevation and/or significant Q waves. Then use the infarction squares to determine the type of infarction. For example, if there were ST elevation in leads II, III, aVF, and V_5 and V_6, you would note that the MI involves inferior and lateral leads. The MI would be inferior-lateral.

I Lateral	**aVR** Ignore this lead when looking for MIs	**V₁** Anterior (posterior if mirror image)	**V₄** Anterior
II Inferior	**aVL** Lateral	**V₂** Anterior (posterior if mirror image)	**V₅** Lateral
III Inferior	**aVF** Inferior	**V₃** Anterior	**V₆** Lateral

MI Criteria

Location of MI	EKG Changes	Coronary Artery
Anterior	Indicative changes in V_1 to V_4 Reciprocal changes in II, III, aVF	Left anterior descending (LAD)
Inferior	Indicative changes in II, III, aVF Reciprocal changes in I, aVL, and V leads	Right coronary artery (RCA)
Lateral	Indicative changes in I, aVL, V_5 to V_6 May see reciprocal changes in II, III, aVF	Circumflex
Posterior	No indicative changes, since no leads look directly at posterior wall Diagnosed by reciprocal changes in V_1 and V_2 (large R wave, upright T wave, and possibly ST depression), seen as a mirror image of an anterior MI.	RCA or circumflex
Extensive anterior (sometimes called *extensive anterior-lateral*)	Indicative changes in I, aVL, V_1 to V_6 Reciprocal changes in II, III, aVF	LAD or left main
Anteroseptal	Indicative changes in V_1 and V_2 Usually no reciprocal changes	LAD

Myocardial Infarction Algorithm

This algorithm is designed to point out the myocardial infarction area. Just answer the questions and follow the arrows.

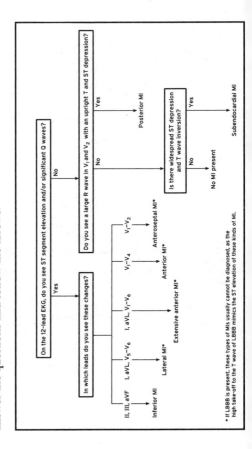

* If LBBB is present, these types of MIs usually cannot be diagnosed, as the high take-off to the T wave of LBBB mimics the ST elevation of these kinds of MI.

Anterior MI Pictorial

An anterior MI damages the front (anterior) wall of the left ventricle. It is a large MI. Look for EKG changes in leads V_1 to V_4.

I	aVR	V_1	V_4
II	aVL	V_2	V_5
III	aVF	V_3	V_6

This is an **acute anterior MI,** as evidenced by the ST elevation in V_1 to V_4. Also note the reciprocal ST depression in leads II, III, and aVF.

If this MI were **age indeterminate,** it would have more normal ST segments, significant Q waves, and T wave inversions in V_1 to V_4.

If this MI were **old,** it would have only the significant Q wave remaining. The ST segment would be back at baseline and the T wave would be upright.

Inferior MI Pictorial

An inferior MI damages the bottom (inferior) wall of the left ventricle. Look for EKG changes in leads II, III, and aVF.

This is an **acute inferior MI.** Note the ST elevation in leads II, III, and aVF. Note also the reciprocal ST segment depression in leads I, aVL, and V_1 to V_6.

The **age indeterminate inferior MI** would have more normal ST segments along with significant Q waves and inverted T waves in leads II, III, and aVF.

The **old inferior MI** would have only significant Q waves in II, III, and aVF. The ST segments would be at baseline and T waves would be upright.

Lateral MI Pictorial

Lateral wall MIs damage the left side wall (lateral wall) of the left ventricle. Look for EKG changes in leads I, aVL, and V_5 and V_6.

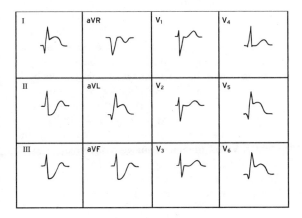

This is an **acute lateral wall MI,** as evidenced by the ST elevation in leads I, aVL, and V_5 to V_6. Note also the reciprocal ST depression in leads II, III, and aVF.

If this were an **age indeterminate lateral MI,** there would be more normal ST segments along with significant Q waves and inverted T waves in I, aVL, and V_5 to V_6.

An **old lateral wall MI** would have baseline ST segments, significant Q waves, and upright T waves in I, aVL, and V_5 to V_6.

Posterior MI Pictorial

Posterior MIs damage the back (posterior) wall of the left ventricle. Since we don't routinely put EKG leads on the back, we are not able to see a posterior MI in the same way as other MIs. With other MIs, we look directly at the damaged area by way of the leads placed directly over that area. For posterior MIs, we look through the front of the heart to see the back. It's rather like looking through the front of a cola bottle to see the very back. What we'd see on the front is the mirror image of what's on the back. For other types of MIs, we look for ST elevation, Q waves, and inverted T waves. For posterior MIs, we look for big R waves (the mirror image of a Q wave), ST depression (the mirror image of ST elevation), and upright T waves (the mirror image of inverted T waves). Look for these EKG changes in V_1 and V_2.

Posterior MIs almost always accompany an inferior MI, so always look in leads II, III, and aVF for the inferior MI.

Posterior MI Pictorial (con't)

This is an **acute posterior wall MI.** Note the tall R wave in V_1 to V_2 along with ST segment depression and an upright T wave. Note that there is an acute inferior MI as well.

An **age indeterminate posterior MI** would have more normal ST segments, a tall R wave, and an upright T wave.

The **old posterior MI** would have only the tall R wave remaining. The ST segments would be at baseline and the T wave would be inverted.

Extensive Anterior MI Pictorial (Also Called Extensive Anterior-Lateral MI)

An extensive anterior MI is a huge, often catastrophic, MI. It damages the anterior and lateral walls of the left ventricle. Look for EKG changes in leads I, aVL, and V_1 to V_6.

Here we have a huge MI, the **acute extensive anterior MI.** Note the ST elevation in I, aVL, and V_1 to V_6 and the reciprocal ST depression in II, III, and aVF.

The **age indeterminate extensive anterior MI** would have more normal ST segments along with significant Q waves and T wave inversion.

The **old extensive anterior MI** would have baseline ST segments, significant Q waves, and upright T waves in I, aVL, and V_1 to V_6.

Anteroseptal MI Pictorial

An anteroseptal MI is a small MI that damages only the part of the anterior wall that includes the septum. Look for EKG changes in leads V_1 and V_2.

This is an **acute anteroseptal MI.** Note the ST elevation in leads V_1 to V_2.

An **age indeterminate anteroseptal MI** would have more normal ST segments, significant Q waves, and inverted T waves in V_1 to V_2.

The **old anteroseptal MI** would have only significant Q waves remaining in V_1 to V_2. The ST segments would be at baseline and the T waves would be upright.

Subendocardial MI Pictorial

A subendocardial MI is an MI that damages only the thin innermost layer of the myocardium. It is a small MI that usually progresses within a few months to a full-thickness MI if treatment is not rendered. A subendocardial MI is a type of non–Q wave MI. Look for widespread EKG changes throughout the 12-lead EKG.

This is an **acute subendocardial MI.** It is characterized by widespread ST depression and T wave inversions. Subendocardial infarctions are diagnosed only in the acute phase, as they do not cause significant Q waves, and their T waves are already inverted.

Lead Placement for a Right-Sided EKG

A right-sided EKG is done with the limb leads in their normal places, but with the precordial leads placed on the right side of the chest instead of the left. Right-sided EKGs are used to diagnose right ventricular infarctions.

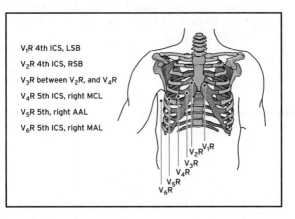

V_1R 4th ICS, LSB

V_2R 4th ICS, RSB

V_3R between V_2R, and V_4R

V_4R 5th ICS, right MCL

V_5R 5th, right AAL

V_6R 5th ICS, right MAL

Right Ventricular Infarction (Right-Sided EKG)

Right ventricular infarctions are not as common as MIs that affect the left ventricle. When seen, right ventricular infarctions accompany an inferior wall MI. Right ventricular infarctions are recognized by ST segment elevation in right-sided EKG leads V_3R or V_4R. A standard EKG, which looks at the left ventricle, will not pick up a right ventricular infarction.

On this right-sided EKG, note the ST elevation in leads V_3R to V_4R. This proves there is an RV infarction. You'll note also that there is ST elevation in leads II, III, and aVF that indicate an inferior MI. Remember, the right-sided EKG leaves the limb leads in their normal place, but moves the precordial leads to the right side of the chest. So the inferior MI will still be obvious on the right-sided EKG.

Pericarditis

Pericarditis is an inflammation of the pericardial sac, the sac that surrounds the heart. The myocardial layer just beneath this inflamed pericardium also becomes inflamed, causing temporary EKG changes that can mimic the changes seen with an acute MI. Pericarditis is recognized by widespread concave ST elevation.

I	aVR	V_1	V_4
II	aVL	V_2	V_5
III	aVF	V_3	V_6

Note the widespread concave ST elevation in leads I, II, III, aVL, aVF, and V_1 to V_6. This is *not* typical of an MI because it is so widespread. Is it possible this is a huge MI instead of pericarditis? Sure. But based on the concave ST elevation scattered across many leads, it's more likely that it's pericarditis. Only by examining the patient would we know for sure.

Early Repolarization

Early repolarization is a variation of a normal EKG. Repolarization begins so early in this condition that the T wave appears to start before the QRS has even finished. This makes it look like the ST segment is slightly elevated, mimicking an MI. There is often a "fishhook" at the end of some QRS complexes that gives a hint that there is early repolarization.

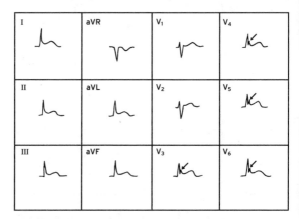

In this EKG, note the mild ST segment elevation in almost all leads and the fishhook in V_3 to V_6 (see arrows). This is typical of early repolarization.

Miscellaneous EKG Effects

Effect	EKG Change
Digitalis effect	Prolonged PR interval, sagging ST segment depression
Quinidine effect	Prolonged QT interval, wide T wave
Hyperkalemia	Tall, pointy T waves
Severe hyperkalemia	Widened QRS complex
Hypokalemia	Flattened T wave, prominent U wave
Hypercalcemia	Shortened, almost nonexistent, ST segment
Hypocalcemia	Prolonged ST segment, causing prolonged QT interval

Index